HERBAL CURES OF DUODENAL ULCER AND GALL STONES

This book has been written so that sufferers from duodenal ulcers and gall stones can better understand their complaint and set about the curing of it once and for all.

GW00645508

Herbal Cures of Duodenal Ulcer and Gall Stones

by

Frank Roberts

(Member of The National Institute of Medical Herbalists)
Diploma of Botano-Therapy

ATHENE PUBLISHING CO. LTD.
Wellingborough, Northamptonshire

First published 1952
Seventh Edition 1969
Third Impression 1972
Eighth Edition 1975
Second Impression 1977
Third Impression 1978
Fourth Impression 1981

ISBN 0 7225 0284 2

Printed in Great Britain by
Lowe and Brydone (Printers) Ltd., Bramley, Leeds,
and bound by Weatherby Woolnough,
Wellingborough, Northamptonshire.

To

MY WIFE

who has helped so much in the preparation of my manuscripts and who was such a cheery and welcoming receptionist before I retired from private practice.

Contents

Preface to the Eighth Edition

It is now twenty-two years since this book was first published. During these years it has found its way into nearly every country in the world and some hundreds of thousands, with pending operations cancelled, have been cured by having taken the simple treatment that is presented.

For a long spell the demand exceeded the supply. Sufferers could not find any herbalists able to dispense the liquids or make the tablets to the same formula. But the position has altered since then. Although the liquid is still hard to find, the tablets are made and held by most herbalists — and so are the tablets covering the gall stones prescription in the second part of this book. Herbalists would almost certainly be able to procure and mix the powders for you if they do not hold the manufactured tablets. They are free to do so because there is no such thing as a 'patent medicine' or secret formula nowadays. Published prescriptions can be prepared and sold by anyone. This fact has given me real satisfaction because I have always adhered to the principle of 'the greatest good to the greatest number'. If your own local herbalist cannot supply the tablets (the liquid being almost unobtainable) then you are invited to write direct, with a stamped-addressed envelope, to Frank Roberts (Herbal Dispensaries) Ltd., 91 Newfoundland Road, Bristol BS2 9LT).

Every type of persons has reported full cure,

from the brain-worker and executive to the shift-worker on the railways, from professional men and women to the phlegmatic workers on the farms and in the docks and on the roads. This treatment knows no such thing as class-distinction — nor colour-bar, nor limitations of age. Youngsters of eighteen as well as octogenarians have completely cleared the disease within the six months.

My real regret is that this well-proven treatment has not yet been brought into the National Health Service and made freely available to the public. How many thousands of hospital beds could have been left available for more serious and intractable diseases! How many countless hours of doctors' time could have been saved (together with unbelievable quantities of various chemicals and pain-killing drugs!) — and with a treatment that is virtually trouble-free except when the frequently associated disease of gall-stones co-exists.

These aspects, as well as the facts in this book, should influence the orthodox medical profession to carry through intensive testings and *provings* that will lead to this simple and harmless treatment being accepted as an official one that can be prescribed under the National Health Service by any doctor and with all pharmacists being able to dispense it in both liquid and tablet form.

I present to you the information in these pages with even more confidence than when it first appeared twenty-two years ago.

January 1975

Preface to the First Edition

This book was written at the suggestion of the well-known composer and writer on unorthodox medicine, Mr Cyril Scott. After reading through a very lengthy manuscript of mine on the treatment of nearly every known digestive disease, Mr Scott singled out the duodenal ulcer treatment as something which ought to be given a book to itself.

The original 'Duodenal Ulcer Cure' chapter was eleven pages long. It was concise and to the point. However, one chapter in a book of nearly thirty chapters could not fully cover the whole subject or convey the unbounded confidence with which I present this treatment to the general public . . . and all sufferers from this common disease want to know *everything* possible about their trouble.

Apart from this, a book containing every digestive disease is quite a volume, and such volumes cost a lot of money nowadays. So why should a D.U. sufferer have to buy a large, expensive book when he can get far more information about the disease and its cure from an inexpensive publication like this present one?

Here you have that chapter extended out of all knowledge and made available as a pocket-book at what publishers call 'a popular price'.

March 1952

Introduction

This book has not been written for practitioners. It has carefully avoided every kind of technicality so that the tens of thousands of duodenal ulcer sufferers in this country can understand their own disease and set about the curing of it once and for all.

If you are not a practitioner it means that you are reading these words for one of three good reasons:—

(1) You have a duodenal ulcer; you know it because it has been proved beyond a shadow of a doubt. (In which case I would assure you that your disease *can* be cured with medicine — herbal medicine — and the following pages will tell you how.)

OR

(2) Someone who means a lot to you has a duodenal ulcer. (In which case you can put an end to his or her suffering by insisting that the treatment and advice in this book should be taken.)

OR

(3) You have a shrewd idea that you have a duodenal ulcer, but you are afraid to tell your doctor about it and have your worst fears realized. (In which case I would advise you to go carefully through the symptoms as given in Chapter 8. If you have eighty per cent of those symptoms of an advanced case, then you have such an ulcer. This applies even though your

duodenal ulcer does not yet reveal itself on any X-ray plate. Treat yourself as suggested in these pages and your trouble will be brought to an end.)

Does all this sound too good to be true, too confident? Perhaps it does! However, I am not offering you a lot of unproved theories; I have personally treated very many thousands of duodenal ulcer patients along these simple lines, and the record of complete and X-ray-proofed cures would stagger the orthodox medicos who soothe the ulcer with bismuth, chlorodyne, belladonna and similar prescriptions until the patient is compelled to go into hospital for surgery or a temporary 'patching up' with a diet. The sceptic will immediately ask the obvious question: 'If this treatment is so effective, why don't the doctors prescribe it?' The simple answer is that the doctors can only prescribe those remedies which appear in the two volumes known as the *British Pharmacopoeia* and the *British Pharmaceutical Codex*. Two of the herbal ingredients in the basic formula do not appear in either of these books; it is therefore impossible for a doctor to write a prescription to cover the complete formula: and even if you 'wangled' this prescription, there is no pharmacist who would have those two ingredients which would allow him to dispense the complete formula. The medical herbalists are the only ones who would be holding the ingredients in their dispensaries as things are at present.

Some of the most successful duodenal ulcer cures have been those of patients who began the treatment as out-and-out sceptics who had no faith in the prescribed formula; it all seemed too simple to be effective. This therefore rules out any suggestion that 'faith healing' enters into the treatment.

Are you still sceptical? Probably you are. So, before you begin with Chapter One, let me present you to another sceptic, Mr N.S., of Bradford, Yorks. He wrote to me as follows:

> Your claim about curing an ulcer seems too good to be true. However, I naturally hope that it is all you claim it to be because I have just had an X-ray at the Bradford Royal Infirmary and one of the specialists there informs me that I definitely have a *chronic* duodenal ulcer which, in his opinion, can *not* be cured by treatment.

He took the treatment and sent me the following letter three months later (i.e., before his treatment had been completed):

> I have been successful in my application for a further X-ray examination at the Infirmary and have been to see the specialist this afternoon to get the result. I am very pleased (which is putting it mildly!) to say that he informed me that my ulcer is cured — which is no mean achievement for a definite chronic duodenal ulcer. However, I can now recommend your treatment not just with confidence but with the definite assurance and proof in my own personal experience with X-ray verification.

Finally, let me answer another question that worries sufferers before they take this treatment: '*Is the cure permanent?*'

I can best answer this by referring you to the very first patient who was treated with the full five-remedy treatment in 1946 (before which the post-war shortages had compelled me to treat patients over a longer period of months with only three of the ingredients). In 1967 Mr E.N.S. of Southport, Lancashire wrote:

> I have intended writing you for some time now to express

my pleasure and gratitude for the wonderful cure that I obtained from your medications for the most painful and distressing illness I was sufferng from for years and which had in 1946 become so acute that I was having haemorrhage every few weeks and lived in dread of a recurrence daily.

I had been operated upon for duodenal ulcer in 1936, but within two years I had a return of the pain and eventually the haemorrhage.

Within three weeks of beginning to take your medications I was free from pain and now, after fifteen years, I have lost the fear of haemorrhage and I am able to eat most things that would have normally made me very ill.

Since 1946 I have been visited by *dozens* of people who have heard of my wonderful improvement in health, and, as you will no doubt be aware, I have put them in touch with you and they have *all* received cure of their awful pain and discomfort.

Once more let me express my warmest gratitude for my return to normal health — and I shall continue to send all and sundry to you as long as they keep coming.

With best wishes for your continued success.

So please drop that scepticism. Procure the treatment — and CURE YOURSELF.

1. What is a Duodenal Ulcer?

Briefly, a duodenal ulcer is an open sore in the tube which leads out of the stomach. This tube is roughly horsehoe shaped and it begins at the lower side of the stomach valve (called the pylorus). In length the duodenum is about twelve fingers' breadths — hence its name (from the Latin *duodeni*, 'twelve together'); call it ten inches long and you won't be far out. The duodenum ends where the small intestine proper begins at the jejunum. The head of the pancreas fits into the concave part of the horseshoe; at about the centre of this concave part, a common duct from the liver, gall bladder and pancreas empties its combined juices into the duodenum.

Duodenal ulcer is essentially a twentieth-century disease. For instance, Dr John M. Scudder's thirteenth edition of *The Eclectic Practice of Medicine* was published in 1891. It contains over 800 fair sized pages and just about covers every known disease. But it contains no reference whatever to duodenal ulcer. On going forward only twenty-eight years we find the following in the 1919 edition of Power's *The Practitioner's Surgery*:

> Duodenal ulcer is *a common disease*. It is only lately that this truth has become generally recognised. In earlier days many patients presenting the symptoms which we now know to be caused by duodenal ulceration were said to be suffering from 'functional disorders', 'acid gastritis', 'hyperchlorhydria', etc., and the

discrimination between gastic and duodenal ulcers had not been appreciated. We now realise that duodenal ulcer is approximately *twelve times as frequent as gastric ulcer*, as judged by cases seen upon the operating table.

Since Dr Power wrote these words over half-a-century has gone by — and in my own experience I find that there are now about one hundred duodenal ulcers to every one gastric ulcer.

The two World Wars seem to have had a lot to do with the increase of these ulcers. It was one year after the First World War that Dr Power stated that 'duodenal ulcer is now a common disease'. Since the Second World War the incidence of this disease has again multiplied on itself to an alarming extent — so much so that I have even had young people, male and female, of seventeen, eighteen and nineteen years of age with fully developed ulcers.

The disease is now so wide-spread and common that it must be a source of concern to physicians and surgeons alike.

2.   Surgery Cannot Cure an Ulcer

When I was a very young man I had a chance to see a duodenal ulcer develop and run its course over the years until it eventually killed the patient. The sufferer was my own father.

My father was a cheerful man. When I was a lad he enjoyed life to the full and had that suggestion of plumpness which seems to go hand-in-hand with a happy outlook. He was not the type of man who is normally subject to internal ulcers, but maybe his responsible position and conscientiousness did more harm than his 'off-duty' cheerfulness could undo. Anyway, the ulcer revealed itself suddenly. One day he was his usual self. The next day he was feeling very off-colour; and on the same evening he had a severe haemorrhage. He was rushed to hospital and an emergency operation took place. After a few weeks he was home again. He had been told that the operation was a complete success. But he had lost a lot of weight, and he never regained it. Although the operation was 'a success', he could not eat the normal diet of pre-operation days. He was on a strict diet from then onwards. If the operation had been the success that was claimed, then the conservative diet should have prevented any remote possibility of a recurrence — and he ought not to have started feeling the ulcer pains again within a month or two of the operation. Eventually there was a bursting of the 'successfully' cleared ulcer. The haemorrhage was so severe this time that he died before he could be rushed to the hospital for another operation.

The above will explain why I have always been so sincerely interested in a virtually infallible medicinal treatment and cure of duodenal ulcer.

Dangers of Suppressive Treatment

A surgical operation *cannot* cure an ulcer. Despite their great learning and accomplishments, the physicians and surgeons are extremely illogical in their approach to certain bodily conditions. For instance, the orthodox treatment of skin diseases assumes that the trouble lies there on the surface; just rub ointments in and try to clear it; if the skin is hot or inflamed, swab it with calamine lotion. But the skin with a rash, etc., on it is not the same as a lump of rock covered with patches of moss. There is blood coursing through every minutest pinpoint area of the skin — and the skin is one of the parts of the body which eliminates unwanted fluids and poisons from the blood. Also, as the blood comes both *to* and *from* every cell of the skin, the blood and lymph going away from a diseased spot is carrying specks of poison from it into the blood stream. Therefore, whether the skin disease is due to the body eliminating poisons or to an external infection (due to, say, dirt getting in a small scratch), the only safe and sure way of getting to the root of the trouble is by the taking of medicine which will clear the blood of its present impurities. Any suppressive treatment with only an ointment or lotion is forcing the surface poisons to go down into the deeper tissues; when the surface is cleared, everything may look fine — but it won't take long before those buried poisons multiply up and are thrown up to the surface in a skin disease of greater severity than the original one.

Now if the orthodox approach is illogical in respect of the vast range of skin diseases, may we not look for a bit of wrong thinking where *other* diseases are concerned? Looking at it from the surgical angle, will the cutting out of a boil cure the condition? What happens to all the poisons which have already been carried from the boil and around the system by the ever-flowing blood? Similarly with a duodenal ulcer (which is in effect a 'boil' on a wet internal membrane); your system has chosen that duodenal spot as the place from which body poisons shall discharge. The surgeon cuts out the ulcer; the operation is a 'success' — but what happens to all the other poisons which were flowing to and from the ulcer at the time when the ulcer was cut out? Those poisons are still in the system and they want to get out. The duodenal membrane is made to heal over by the surgeon — but the system of that particular patient insists that the poisons outlet shall always be in the duodenum, and nothing will divert them elsewhere. So, for a variable time, the patient feels better. But, during this time, the poisons are again being deposited in the lower layers of the duodenal membrane and gradually eating themselves upwards to the surface. And when they break through again, there is the ulcer on the same spot and just as bad and painful as ever it was despite the 'successful' operation.

3. Chemicals and Poisons Cannot Cure an Ulcer

The orthodox medicinal treatment of duodenal ulcer is a rather feeble effort, as I think you will agree when you have read this chapter.

The general idea is to reduce the pain. In a way this is a laudable aim. But it is not enough; and the *suppressing* of pain and symptoms can be very dangerous. For instance . . .

The usual orthodox medicine for duodenal ulcer is bismuth, belladonna and chlorodyne. The bismuth is not meant to be absorbed into the system. It is swallowed so that it can form a shield over the ulcer. The bismuth keeps depositing its particles upon the ulcer; when the deposit is thick enough, the ulcer is shielded from the painful friction of the food moving out of the stomach and through the duodenum. While the 'plating' of bismuth is being formed, it is the job of the chlorodyne and belladonna to inhibit the pain. When the bismuth shield is formed, the chlorodyne and belladonna are often left out of the subsequent prescriptions.

So this treatment has reached the stage when the ulcer is lying under a plate of caked bismuth particles. Now the bismuth has no ability to kill off the ulcer poisons — nor have any of the three ingredients (or any other similar additions that I know) the power to destroy or eliminate poisons in the blood stream or the tissues. And so the whole line of treatment fails to get within a hundred miles of a cure. It merely puts off the evil day when the surgeon has to take a hand in things. Here is what happens . . .

You have a plating of hard bismuth over your ulcer. The ulcer is *growing* beneath this shield. Either it can bore 'backwards' and perforate the external membrane of the duodenum — in which case it is an immediate surgical case. Or the ulcer can remain shallow but increase in its surface area; this would mean that the bismuth shield would also increase in area; but, when you remember the shape of the duodenum, you will find that this shield is a concave one which is enlarging on two curved surfaces which lie in different planes — and the circumference of such a concave circle has to reach a limit beyond which it starts breaking up and throwing cracks across the entire shield: the friction of food rubs away pieces of the broken plating, and the ulcer is again exposed, much bigger than before and probably bleeding as well as discharging pus. So the long-suffering patient is passed to the surgeon; there is a 'successful' operation, and soon the whole cycle begins all over again.

Biochemic Preparation of Body Salts

There is another good reason why chemicals and poisons cannot effect a cure. The cure *must* be brought about by clearing the ulcer where it lies *and also by clearing every tissue of the body of the poisons that will otherwise seep out and gravitate towards the duodenum.* Poisons cannot clean out poisons; by definition, poisons are things which are able to kill off body cells — and dead body cells merely mean more debris and poisons let loose in the system. Crude chemicals are unable to enter into the actual body cells; therefore unhealthy cells remain unhealthy. (It is this shortcoming of crude chemicals that brought about the biochemical system of medicine; in this system the body salts needed by the cells are prepared homoeopathically: a body cell can only 'eat' solitary molecules: crude chemicals always consist of huge masses of molecules all stuck together — and even the particles of the finest chemical powder are actually huge bunches of adhering molecules which the cells cannot absorb. The biochemic preparation is made by hours and hours of grinding each salt into an overwhelming mass of sugar or milk; the final product contains isolated molecules such as we find in the juices of fruits and vegetables and other foods; these important and essential body salts can thus be made to enter the actual cells so that the cells are fully nourished and strong enough to expel any unwanted impurities. Crude chemicals might be compared with super-colossal locomotives which can get as far as the destination but are too huge to get inside the station, thus rendering the whole journey null and void.)

4. Diet is Not a Satisfactory Answer

I have the utmost respect for dietetics as one of the sciences of health. However, my own idea of a *curative* dietetic treatment is one which will allow the patient to revert to enjoyable meals again after the diet has accomplished its work. Put it this way: if I gave a medicinal ulcer treatment to a patient and then expected him to go on a diet which he finds unpalatable for perhaps the rest of his life, I should consider the treatment very unconvincing and unsatisfactory. Yet this is the usual dietetic attitude to ill health, and it is little wonder that sufferers look for an alternative which gives them the hope of reverting to the foods which tickle their palates and make up quite a part of the contentment with — and enjoyment of — life.

Eating what you like keeps you happy — and keeping yourself happy is one of the best ways of keeping yourself healthy. If sickness comes to you (as it does to everyone — yes, even those who are on a diet to prevent illness), then you are undoubtedly advised to adjust your diet until you are cured. When you are *cured* you should be able to revert to the foods you were eating before you became ill. I am afraid that I cannot bring myself to be dogmatic or narrow-minded on the subject of diet when a person is in health; there are so many schools of thought on the subject: here are three startling examples: Dr Salisbury's diet consisted of meat, meat, meat and *nothing* but meat. The vegetarians cut out all meats and so-called 'animal foods'. The vegans go one further and take a poor view of the orthodox vegetarians because they drink milk and eat eggs, cheese, honey, etc., which are all animal products because they are obtained from animal life.

Bland Diet Cannot Cure

In treating duodenal ulcers with diet it is possible to eat such a bland and non-irritant diet that the food always runs smoothly past the ulcer without any painful friction and actually allows a certain amount of self-healing of the ulcer to go forward. But this progress reaches a certain stage and then stops. The proof of this lies in the fact that the remainder of the ulcer will soon liven up and give trouble if you suddenly and radically alter this diet; and this will 'happen even though the patient has been on the bland diet for a very long time previously. Another proof of the non-curative pretensions of the bland diet is the fact that so many patients have told me at their first interview that they have been informed that they will possibly have to remain on their 'slop' diet *for the rest of their lives* — and I don't blame them for shuddering at the prospect.

Diet may have completely cured an odd case here and there. In such a case the ulcer would not have had time to seriously impair the self-curative resistance of the body. The diet has then allowed the ulcer to lie quiet and undisturbed whilst the system clears itself of *all* the ulcer poisons (this being the only way in which any full cure can be achieved. — i.e., by complete elimination of every speck of ulcer infection throughout the organism). However, I have still to be convinced that a diet will *cure* ulcers of twenty years' standing; and yet the herbal medicinal treatment given in this book has cured many such cases within three to four months and allowed these chronic sufferers to revert to a full and varied diet which they have now, in several cases, been enjoying for years without any trouble or signs of a recurrence.

5. Using Your Own Self-Curative Powers

This chapter has nothing to do with auto-suggestion or anything else which has to be self-administered. Self-repair and self-cure are two of the survival factors which are 'keyed-in' to every form of animal life. You can accelerate these processes with the right line of treatment, or you can hinder and inhibit them with a treatment which pulls in opposite directions to these two forces.

These two forces are considered as one factor in both herbalism and homoeopathy. The term 'Vital Force' covers this inherent power of the body to repair and cure itself.

There are many things about the 'Vital Force' which are now established as facts.

For instance:

1. The Vital Force is able to cure all acute diseases without other assistance. (An acute disease is one which flares up suddenly and can be mild or severe.)

2. The Vital Force needs help in the cure of chronic diseases. (These are diseases which have slowly, insidiously and firmly established themselves in the body and have been maintaining a slight lead over the power of the Vital Force to catch up with the rate of deterioration.)

3. The Vital Force always acts from the centre outwards.

4. The Vital Force is selective and cures the organs and functions in the order of their

importance.

These are the most important activities of the Vital Force and are sufficient for the consideration of duodenal ulceration. Of these, Rule 3 looks the most vague and unimportant — and yet it is the Master Rule for our present purposes. Your cure *must* come from the centre outwards — i.e., self-cure insists that your duodenal ulcer is a surface manifestation and is an out-thrusting of poisons which are being driven out of the deep tissues by the Vital Force. (To get the angle on this, you are reminded that the *inner* membrane of the duodenum is actually an *external* surface of the body. The whole of the digestive tract from the mouth down through to the anus is a hollow tube, and the surfaces of that tube are the inner limits reached by the tissues (just as the skin represents the outer limits.) Take a rough cross-section through the body like this:

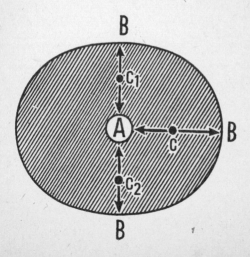

The small circle is the cross-section of the digestive tract. All the shaded part is 'you'. Parts A and B are not 'you' — 'A' being merely a hole, and 'B' being the air around you. Therefore the *centre* of your tissues would be at such points as C, C_1 and C_2 — and the Vital Force would act in two directions, from C outwards to B, and from C *out*wards to the surface of A.

Now if your self-curative power is moving your poisons both to the ulcer and from the ulcer, any treatment which directly attacks the ulcer and ignores the residue of the trouble which is moving from C outwards to B will never effect a cure.

Our curative treatment must therefore fully cover the hidden half of your trouble (the C to B half) which is not taken into account by treatment with surgery, chemicals or poisons. And it is mainly on this aspect of the Vital Force that diet treatment is a long-term failure; the body needs protein, fats, carbohydrates, food containing all necessary tissue salts, water, and vitamins — and these have to be eaten (or drunk) in variety and quantity that ensures that they reach the tissues in the approximate percentages that mean healthy eating and allow the Vital Force to function at maximum efficiency. Putting it more simply, a severely restricted diet lowers the Vital Force and this lowers your ability to achieve self-cure.

6. Choosing the Curative Remedies

In the herbal therapy there are very many hundreds of powerful and harmless remedies. Nearly all of them have composite therapeutic properties. Take a well-known one, witch hazel; it is astringent *and* discutient *and* tonic *and* stimulating *and* aromatic, etc. (The 'etc.' represents other properties which develop when witch hazel is heated). So our problem is to choose from all available remedies the minimum number which will cover every curative aspect of duodenal ulceration and yet exclude every unwanted therapeutic activity.

Before we can choose remedies we ought to know more about the cause of the ulcer.

Basic Cause of Ulcer

What causes the ulcer to form? Opinions vary, but my own theory is that the basic cause is worry and/or hurry and/or fatigue that results in chronic contraction of the duodenal membrane and which also affects the stomach so that there is a seepage of gastric acid through the valve (pylorus) into the duodenum. Now the duodenum is an *alkaline* area of the digestive tract, whereas the stomach is an *acid* area. If free stomach acid seeps in fair quantities into the duodenum it is possible for the alkaline condition to become neutralized and for the excess acid to make the duodenum into an *acid* area — this being an abnormal condition which would tend to corrode the tense membrane and initiate an ulcer. The treatment is formulated to rectify these assumed conditions, and the results achieved would seem to prove the correctness of the theory. Even if it is suggested that it seems unnatural for a body secretion to corrode a membrane, then the alternative suggestion is that the abnormality of an *acid* condition in an *alkaline* area would set up spasms in that area; and if a spasm is maintained over a long period the tissue cells in that area become undernourished and weakened; with the membrane now reduced to an unnatural condition there is nothing unnatural in a body acid proving itself too potent for the weakened membrane. The incipient ulcer is there as soon as the first tissue cells are corroded, and the poisons from these dead cells multiply where they lie and are also carried around the system by the blood washing past the area.

Looking for deeper causes, we find the case of the system which has developed an excess of normal impurities and wishes to discharge them from the body. If the skin is reasonably healthy but the duodenal membrane is abnormal (as in the case above), then the poisons will be thrown towards the duodenum and discharged into it instead of running to the skin and forming boils or some suppurating skin disease.

The Lymphatic System

So first we ought to make the body kill off its own poisons *internally*. We have inside us a wonderful scavenging system for doing this work; it is called the lymphatic system, and, when working properly, it takes care of the destruction of all poisons. Have you ever felt an enlarged gland in your armpit when some part of your hand or arm has become septic? That is one of many lympathic glands doing its work, charging itself with poison from the septic area and breaking it all down into its harmless components. The one herbal remedy which stimulates the whole of the lymphatic system is echinacea; this is our first remedy.

Next, the nervous tightness (spasm) in the duodenal membrane; also, the inhibited action of the goblet glands in the affected area and the sub-activity of other glands in the body. Poke root covers all this and becomes our second ingredient.

Next, we have the urgent job of soothing the ulcer and preventing any further 'decay' at the site of the ulcer. Here we can safely choose marshmallow root; for centuries this has been called Mortification Root because of its power to halt the mortification of ulcerous tissue. This is our third remedy.

American Golden Seal

Next we must see to it that the cells of the membrane are revitalized. We must also regulate the flow and seepage of gastric acid. We must also cover any damage or impairment of the functions of every other part of the digestive system. This is a tall order and calls for a rather special remedy. It is American golden seal. Not only is golden seal the superlative vitalizer and normalizer of the digestive tract, but it has the strange property of being able to magnify the therapeutic activities of all the other remedies which are mixed with it. (I ought to mention that this extract is imported, it is in short supply and it is expensive. And whilst on this matter of cost, I can give you a pointer to the inclusive outlay on this treatment — it costs about the same as the average duodenal ulcer sufferer spends on alkaline powder in one year!) Golden seal is our fourth remedy.

Lastly we have to gently astringe the duodenal membrane so that the lax tissues that have fallen away around the ulcer are gently tightened and eventually knitted healthily and scarlessly together again. To halt and prevent bleeding of the ulcer we also need a styptic. Cranesbill root covers these requirements and becomes our fifth and last remedy.

Some medical herbalists vary the above ingredients. However, the exact reasons for the choice of these particular ingredients are given above and I cannot conceive of any improvement upon this thoroughly proven formula. (Homoeopathic sulphur 6x pilules — one part sulphur in one million of sugar of milk — are sometimes included to make sure that the most obstinate of deep poisons are shifted and eliminated. However, this is a precautionary refinement; the echinacea governs a cleansing system which washes every cell of the body.)

7. Taking the Treatment

THE FORMULA
Tincture of Echinacea — 3½ ounces
Tincture of Poke Root — 3½ ounces
Fluid Extract of Marshmallow Root — 3½ ounces
Fluid Extract of Golden Seal Root — 3½ ounces
Fluid Extract of Cranesbill Root — 3½ ounces

These 17½ ounces of extracts and tinctures constitute the entire treatment and will last you three to four months of continuous medication.

The ingredients are all added together to make one medicine. You simply take three doses of this medicine daily. It all sounds *too* simple, doesn't it? It is the sheer simplicity of the treatment which makes many sufferers scoff at the thought that three or four months of this treatment can do what every other type of treatment has failed to do over periods ranging up to as long as twenty or thirty years. But it is YOUR ulcer and not mine which I am interested in curing, and *you* will be the loser if you pass this treatment by because of its praiseworthy simplicity and speed of cure.

Your dosage of the mixed ingredients is 30 drops in a wineglassful of water three times daily *between* meals — i.e., about two hours after breakfast, lunch and tea. Shake the mixture thoroughly before measuring out each dose or you will get a wrong proportion of the five remedies.

Dietary Restrictions

As regards dietary restrictions, these need apply
only during the first 14 days of your treatment.
During this first fortnight you are advised to cut
all meat and fish out of your diet. *ALL* other
foods are permissible. During these 14 days you
should eat small and frequent meals or snacks,
keep clear of alcoholic drink, and reduce smoking
to the minimum if you happen to be a smoker.
(Trying to give up smoking suddenly and
completely sets up nervous irritability which
hampers the curative progress.) During the third
and fourth weeks of treatment you can gradually
increase the variety and quantity of your diet; all
foods can be included in small but growing
amounts: during this period you should also
reduce the frequency of your snacks until you
bring them back to the normal four meals per
day at normal mealtimes. When you enter the
fifth week of your treatment you should be eating
normal meals at normal mealtimes. (You are
asked to leave the frying-pan alone during the
whole treatment; this is precautionary against
the liver troubles which are often found to have
developed during the life of the ulcer.)

At the end of the fourth week of the treatment
most patients are out of all pain and are eating
well. But this does not mean that the ulcer is fully
cleared at that stage. Do not ease up on your
treatment under any circumstances.

Ensuring Permanancy of Cure

In many cases the patients make very rapid
progress and reach the stage of complete
clearance and healing of the actual ulcer within
the third month. When this happens, the

astringent action of the cranesbill root develops an extra tension of the duodenal membrane and this gives off symptoms which are almost identical to those of the original ulcer. Such patients get the idea that, at this stage, the trouble is still there and just as bad as ever. Actually they are simply receiving signals which indicate that the treatment can be discontinued (or that the cranesbill root is no longer needed). The duodenum may look good and healthy at that stage — but we still have that job of clearing the ulcer poisons throughout all the other tissues of the body. The treatment must therefore go forward to ensure permanancy of cure. The best procedure is to leave off treatment entirely for 48 hours to allow the tightness to die away; then recommence the treatment on *half* doses, at the same three times during each day — and carry on until all the extracts have been taken.

Very occasionally one finds the duodenal ulcer which is complicated by the existence of a second digestive disease. Before covering this matter of complications I must reassure you by stating that my carefully kept records show that only ONE CASE in about 200 has revealed a complication — the others have run a smooth and trouble-free course from start to finish. These odds against your having a complication should put your mind at rest on this point!

Gall Stones

By far the most common *second* digestive disease is gall stones. This is rather to be expected because the outlet of the bile-and-gall duct is actually in the wall of the duodenum. When the horseshoe-shaped duodenum has been made 'puffy' by the inflammation around the ulcer, the aperture in its membranes can be squeezed shut in one of the folds that develops to accommodate the puffiness-expansion of the organ. The bile and gall are held back and transferred to the gall bladder which acts as a reservoir which dehydrates the bile and gall for easy storage. After lots of dehydration the next stage is the formation of solids — i.e., gall stones. (Readers with this complication need have no worry. They should refer to page 42 for full and specific information about the simple treatment whereby the stones will be seen to pass *per rectum* without pain or discomfort within 24 hours, after which a month's treatment will rectify the functions of the gall bladder and clear any inflammation where the stones were lying.).

Any other co-existent digestive diseases or disorders would be of an unimportant nature and would yield readily to simple treatments.

8.   Identifying a Duodenal Ulcer

Are you one of those who think they may have an ulcer but are afraid to know the worst (because you previously thought there was no cure)? If so, here are the symptoms of an advanced case so that you can identify the trouble. The key symptoms are in italics; if you have these key symptoms it is almost certain that you have a duodenal ulcer and you are advised to get in touch with a qualified medical herbalist for probable confirmation and the treatment as given in this book.

The pain can be better described as a distressing discomfort rather than a severe or acute pain. It is of a *gnawing or boring* nature — *a deep, dull ache* with possible local tenderness to the touch. *The time of pain is somewhere around two hours after meals. The pain is relieved very speedily by eating more food.* (When such an ulcer is in its 'infancy', the first discomforts usually come on at about 4 p.m.) *The position of the pain is within a small radius of a point midway between the navel and the lowest point of the breastbone.* The pain sometimes seems to bore through into the back and pain can be felt between the lower parts of the shoulder blades. *There are short periods of fullness* with occasional acid belchings or heartburn. During pain the mouth frequently fills with a tasteless fluid from the salivary glands. Constipation is often present. In severe cases the bowel motions are sometimes tarry-looking. Vomiting is unusual. There is only a limited loss of weight due to the fact that there is no real distaste for food, and eating extra food eases the pain. There is occasional dizziness, especially after stooping. The patient is generally depressed. Many sufferers wake up during the night with 'hunger pains' and have to munch a biscuit or drink a glass of milk to abate the pain.

9. The Treatment and Cure of Gall Stones

Gall Stones have been mentioned as the only likely serious complication (secondary disease) of Duodenal Ulcer. This book would therefore seem to be incomplete without details of the cure referred to on page 38.

Inflammation of the gall bladder usually precedes gall-stone trouble. When gall stones have formed, the condition called cholecystitis (inflammation of the gall bladder) can develop from the lodging of one of the stones in the gall duct. Stone in the duct is the almost invariable cause of acute cholecystitis.

From the above it is obvious that any line of treatment which clears out all stones from the gall bladder and the gall duct will remove the causes of both conditions. Any remaining inflammation will then yield readily to an appropriate formula. If, however, we 'put the cart before the horse' and try to disperse the inflammation before clearing the stones, then no curative headway will be made.

Before going into the details of the diseases and their cure, I would like to make the following clear-cut statement to sufferers from gall stones.

Within twenty-four hours (repeat *hours*) of reading this chapter, you can pass and count all your stones. If you have an operation pending, you are advised to take this simple treatment, wash out the stones from the excrement, take them along to your doctor and inform him that your operation can be cancelled.

What is this remarkable treatment that produces such spectacular results? It is merely olive oil and lemon juice! You may reply that you have already taken a spoonful of olive oil after every meal and an occasional drop of lemon juice, and that your doctor has suggested these remedies, which have achieved nothing. I agree that you could go on like that for ever and still fail to clear your stones. It is no use being half-hearted with these simple but valuable remedies. A pint of the oil will do more in one evening than a hundred pints spread over two or three years. A half-pint of lemon juice taken on that same evening will do more than a thousand lemons could do if spread in small doses over a couple of years. Where orthodoxy is concerned, they have the right remedies but the wrong method.

Treatment Programme

If you want to clear your gall stones by bedtime tomorrow night, buy a pint of purest olive oil and eight or nine lemons. (If lemons are not available, then pure lemon juice, which is now sold in bottled form, will act just as well.) You should commence the treatment at about 7 p.m., and you must be sure not to eat anything after the midday meal on the chosen day (although you can have normal drinks during the interim hours). At about 7 p.m. you take four tablespoonsful of the olive oil and immediately follow them down with one tablespoonful of neat, unsweetened lemon juice. After fifteen minutes, repeat this pair of doses in exactly the same way . . . and continue repeating the pair of doses at intervals of fifteen minutes until all of the oil has been taken; then finish off the treatment by drinking off any remaining lemon juice.

It is important that *all* of the oil should be taken at those fixed intervals and on the same evening. In an occasional case the patient will tend to throw up some of the oil during or after the treatment, and this in spite of the fact that the acid juice 'lays' the oil and takes away the possibility of nausea developing during the treatment. Any oil that may be thrown up is merely an excess quantity which is not required by that particular patient's system for achieving the full results — i.e., the system will either retain and use all of the oil, or else it will use all that it requires and reject the balance. Note carefully: even if you vomit any of the oil during the treatment you must still carry on taking the oil without interfering with the fifteen-minute intervals between doses. If you fail to observe this instruction, it is possible that you may leave stones 'in transit' and these could give biliary colic after a few days, when they begin to move without the soothing, softening action of the oil. No such after-effects have ever come to my knowledge when the full pint of oil has been taken.

What the Stones Look Like

During the twenty-four to forty-eight hours after the taking of this treatment you should pass all bowel motions into a receptacle and run tap water strongly on to the excrement with a view to 'washing out' the stones from it. Most of the stones will sink; some of them may float. When passed per rectum, these stones will be found to be softened to the stage of rubberiness. They may vary from the size of a golf ball to that of a pea or a split pea. In nearly all cases the stones are biliverdin ones — that is to say, they are made of solidified green bile and they are blue-green in appearance. I have only two cases on my files where bilirubin stones were passed. These are stones of solidified red bile pigment, and the patients brought along the stones to me to satisfy my own curiosity. The stones were like strawberries and just as easy to squash between the finger and thumb; mixed with those red stones were others consisting of both green and red bile, the result being stones of the normal colour of gall.

Liquefying Stones

The softening and dissolving action of this treatment is such that it is almost impossible to keep the stones in a bottle for more than about forty-eight hours. The bottled 'souvenirs' will gently fall away into an oily liquid. This leads me on to a possibility which should be mentioned; I refer to the liquefying of stones *before* they are passed per rectum. This happens in very occasional cases, and the result is a needlessly disappointed patient. Such patients will report a very 'messy' series of bowel motions following the treatment. Such patients can be absolutely reassured that everything that was in the gall bladder has been ejected and passed down through the bowel; if any stones were in the gall bladder, they will have come away: it does not matter whether the stones come away in solid or in liquid form provided that you are left with a gall bladder from which every stone and all congested gall have come away. However, such cases of liquefied gall stones are so rare that it is a thousand-to-one chance that you will have the great satisfaction of *seeing your stones* come away after this treatment.

After this simple treatment for overnight clearance of the stones you must take the follow-up treatment for one month to rectify the functions of the gall bladder and disperse inflammation from where the stones were lying. The prescription is made as coated tablets, each tablet containing:—

Pulv. Fringetree	¾ grain
Pulv. Euonymus	¾ grain
Pulv. Kava-Kava	¾ grain
Pulv. Black Root	¾ grain
Pulv. Marshmallow	¾ grain

DOSE:— Two tablets washed down with a little water after every meal.
A minimum of three doses per day must be taken.

During the month of the complete treatment the following foods must be avoided: all fried foods; all fatty and greasy foods; all highly-spiced foods; all pastry and cakes. BUT . . . at the end of the month all of these foods can be gradually brought back into the diet in moderation until a normal full diet is being eaten and enjoyed.

Enquiries to:
Frank Roberts (Herbal Dispensaries) Ltd.,
91 Newfoundland Road,
Bristol BS2 9LT.

Stamped addressed .envelope or International Postal Voucher should be enclosed.

Other recommended books...

MODERN HERBALISM FOR DIGESTIVE DISORDERS
AN ENCYCLOPAEDIA OF NATURAL HEALING

Frank Roberts M.N.I.M.H. Many years in the making, this book gives causes, symptoms, signs and curative prescriptions for digestive ills, including acidosis, alkalosis, appendicitis, constipation, diarrhoea, duodenal ulcer, gall stones, gastric ulcer, liver disorders and stomach troubles. Manner of presentation enables readers to find their ailments quickly and discover their exact treatment and prescription. An outstanding feature is a method whereby suspected diseases can be identified in their early stages. This is a truly comprehensive reference manual to modern practical herbalism for all digestive diseases.

STOMACH ULCERS AND ACIDITY
REMEDIES FOR AVOIDING NEEDLESS PAIN AND SUFFERING

Medical experience over the past twenty-five years indicates that surgical operations for stomach ulcer are useless for curative purposes. Only in extreme cases where the ulcer has eaten a hole through the stomach wall into the peritoneum is surgical treatment warranted. This book explains easily recognized symptoms of ulcer and what causes it. Thirteen therapeutic principles are provided, including restoring the proper acid-alkaline balance of the blood-stream and taking a balanced course of vitamin tablets. The treatment outlined here includes massive doses of vitamin C, which stimulates the formation of scar tissue and causes ulcers to heal rapidly.

SECRETS OF THE CHINESE HERBALISTS
POWERFUL REMEDIES FOR COMMON ILLS

Richard Lucas. *Illustrated.* Fascinating compendium of Chinese herbal remedies for coping with many health problems. Together with herbal recipes that can easily be prepared in your own home this book contains information on certain Oriental herb products sold as fluid extracts, compounds, blends, syrups and ointments, plus a chapter on herbal tonics for adding zest and sparkle to daily living, *and* a chapter on fabulous ginseng, longevity plant, sex rejuvenant, and specific for numerous ailments.

LIVING MEDICINE

THE HEALING PROPERTIES OF PLANTS

Mannfried Pahlow. *8 pages of colour plates.* A guide to plants that have been scientifically proved to have healing properties. Shows how to recognize them, when to pick them, how to prepare them for medicinal use. All the plants and recipes have been especially chosen for use in the home, and are therefore perfectly safe if the instructions are followed exactly. *Includes:* The role of plants in modern medicine; The anatomy of plants; A catalogue of healing plants; The potent, the exotic and the new; Alphabetical home guide to common ailments and corresponding plant remedies.

HERBS: HOW TO GROW AND USE THEM

UNUSUAL TECHNIQUES FOR SUCCESSFUL CULTIVATION

S. I. Khan. *Illustrated.* The author of this concise guide to the successful cultivation of herbs has been growing herbs for many years and has developed some unusual techniques which have been proved to work every time. Here he passes on the fruits of his experience and explains the culinary, cosmetic and medicinal uses of herbs. *Contents include:* Growing and storing herbs; The indoor herb garden; Balconies and roof gardens; Simple hints for drying, storage and freezing; A checklist of common herbs; The herb gardener's year.

INSTANT PAIN CONTROL

TRIGGER POINT SELF-TREATMENT

Leon Chaitow, N.D. *Fully illustrated.* How to locate pain 'triggers' in the body's soft tissue and apply simple self-treatment for easing pain throughout the body. Includes index of symptoms. If pain exists in an area listed there (or in the illustrations), search the appropriate trigger area for a sensitive spot, using thumb or index finger. Once identified as an active trigger, the point should receive up to one minute of sustained or intermittent pressure (or squeezing). This technique can dissipate headache, earache, sinus problems, eye trouble, abdominal pain—any postural, emotional and mechanical stress, or injury.

HERBAL TEAS, TISANES AND LOTIONS

Ceres. *8 pages of full colour plates & over 150 line drawings.* A naturalist describes the many and varied herbs that can be used for making stimulating tonics, soothing infusions and refreshing drinks. She shows how to organize a herb garden to provide tisane, tea and lotion-making herbs, how to make infusions and how to preserve herbs for future use. Apart from their many therapeutic uses, herbal lotions can be used to improve the complexion, add fragrance to bath water, and—as a rinse—impart lustre to the hair.

HOMOEOPATHIC GREEN MEDICINE

Dr. A. C. Gordon Ross. Explains the immense therapeutic potential of some sixty plants, trees and weeds, and their transformation into powerful high-dilution tinctures in the homoeopath's armoury of remedies—without causing injurious side effects. Orthodox medical practitioners also utilize some of these materials, but in a much less efficacious way. Author explains the mistaken orthodox doctrine of isolating, refining and synthesizing the active principle in such plants and makes a plea for a closer liaison between orthodoxy and homoeopathy.

ACUPRESSURE TECHNIQUES
FOR THE SELF-TREATMENT OF MINOR AILMENTS

Dr Hans Ewald. *Illustrated.* Acupressure was developed from the Chinese healing system of acupuncture. It makes use of the same points and meridians (paths), but thumbs and forefingers are used instead of needles. Its prime use is in alleviating and healing nervous diseases, with particular reference to nervous exhaustion, anxiety states, heart and circulatory disturbances, impotence, frigidity, insomnia, headaches, and skin complaints. The technique is explained lucidly in this excellent handbook. Pictures and supplementary drawings indicate the exact location of the points, which should be activated in a clockwise direction for between one and five minutes. Beneficial reaction is quick and lasts for some time.

THE SECRETS OF SUCCESSFUL FASTING

Dr H. Lutzner. When fasting is combined with a specially designed programme of exercise and relaxation, it can be one of the most successful ways to health for people with dietary problems—besides conferring such beneficial side effects as a clear complexion and healthy hair! This book contains something completely new—the first-ever 'do it yourself' guide to a week's fasting, with day-to-day instructions on how to prepare yourself for the treatment and how to look after yourself during it. *Anyone who follows this medically approved programme can be sure of fasting successfully—and without hunger pains!*

THE COMPLETE RAW JUICE THERAPY

Susan E. Charmine. Most comprehensive guide ever published on the healing and regenerative powers of energy-packed raw juices—which contain high concentrations of vitamins, minerals, *natural* sugars and enzymes. When the cells of freshly picked plants are 'unlocked' this goodness is released as pure liquids of great healing value. The gentle action of juices can strengthen the functioning of our bodies and coax them back to normality when they are below par, without risk of side-effects. Author provides an alphabetical list of ailments with exact dosages of appropriate juice remedies and explains exactly how raw juice therapy works.